Herbal Weight Loss Made Simple: Safe, Easy, and Amazing Recipes for Shredding off Unwanted Weight

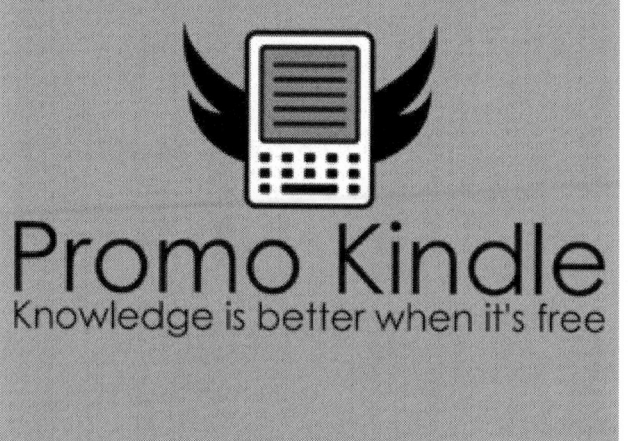

All rights Reserved. No part of this publication or the information in it may be quoted from or reproduced in any form by means such as printing, scanning, photocopying or otherwise without prior written permission of the copyright holder.

Disclaimer and Terms of Use: Effort has been made to ensure that the information in this book is accurate and complete, however, the author and the publisher do not warrant the accuracy of the information, text and graphics contained within the book due to the rapidly changing nature of science, research, known and unknown facts and Internet. The Author and the publisher do not hold any responsibility for errors, omissions or contrary interpretation of the subject matter herein. This book is presented solely for motivational and informational purposes only.

Table of Contents

Adrenal Shocker Smoothie 6

Green Basil Smoothie 7

Blue Mint Smoothie 8

Cilantro Smoothie 9

Ginger Detox Smoothie 10

Green Ginger Smoothie 11

Green Spinach Smoothie 12

Watermelon Smoothie 13

Green Spice Smoothie 14

Mint Chip Smoothie 15

Psoriasis Treatment Smoothie 16

Red Rose Smoothie 17

Hot Fruit Smoothie 18

Green Rose Smoothie 19

Savory Banana Smoothie 20

Anti-Bloat Smoothie 21

Spicy Green Smoothie 22

Strawberry Basil Smoothie 23

Red Mint Fruit Smoothie 24

Red Banana Smoothie 25

Turmeric Tot Smoothie 26

Turmeric Blast Smoothie 27

Sunshine and Turmeric Smoothie 28

Tropics Smoothie 29

Turmeric and Chia Smoothie 30

Adrenal Shocker Smoothie

Ingredients
- 1 C green tea
- ½ avocado
- ½ C blueberries
- ½ T maca
- ½ tsp ginger grated
- ½ T honey
- 1 C kale
- 1 tsp. ginseng

Directions:

I. Add all of your ingredients to your blender or food processor and blend for about 30 seconds on high until smooth
II. Serve

Green Basil Smoothie

Ingredients:
- 1 C coconut water
- 1 banana
- 1 C baby spinach
- basil leaves
- 1 C mixed berries
- 1 T coconut berries
- ¼ tsp cinnamon
- 1 T chia seeds

Directions:
I. Add all of your ingredients to your blender or food processor and blend for about 30 seconds on high until smooth
II. Serve

Blue Mint Smoothie

Ingredients:
- 1 C almond milk
- 1 C blueberries, frozen
- mint leaves
- 1 T chia seeds
- ice
- ½ C frozen raspberries
- 1 S protein powder

Directions:

I. Add all of your ingredients to your blender or food processor and blend for about 30 seconds on high until smooth
II. Serve

Cilantro Smoothie

Ingredients:
- 1 C coconut water
- 1 ice
- 1 banana
- ½ C cilantro
- ½ T coconut oil
- salt
- honey
- 1 C spinach
- ½ mango chunks
- ½ C pineapple chunks

Directions:

I. Add all of your ingredients to your blender or food processor and blend for about 30 seconds on high until smooth
II. Serve

Ginger Detox Smoothie

Ingredients:
- ½ C water
- ½ C medium pulp orange juice
- 1 banana
- ¼ tsp ginger root, grated
- 1 tsp coconut oil
- ½ C pineapple chunks
- ½ C kale

Directions:

I. Add all of your ingredients to your blender or food processor and blend for about 30 seconds on high until smooth
II. Serve

Green Ginger Smoothie

Ingredients:
- 1 C coconut water
- 1 pear, cored
- 1 C baby spinach
- 1 T flaxseed
- 1 tsp coconut oil
- ¼ tsp grated ginger
- ½ T honey
- ½ C frozen mixed berries

Directions:

I. Add all of your ingredients to your blender or food processor and blend for about 30 seconds on high until smooth
II. Serve

Green Spinach Smoothie

Ingredients:
- 1 C coconut water
- 1 C baby spinach
- ½ avocado
- ½ banana
- ½ C blueberries
- ½ T honey
- 1 cored, apple
- 1 coconut flakes

Directions:

I. Add all of your ingredients to your blender or food processor and blend for about 30 seconds on high until smooth
II. Serve

Watermelon Smoothie

Ingredients:
- 1-2 C seeded watermelon
- 1 tsp. grated ginger
- ½ lime, juiced
- ½ C blueberries
- 1 salt
- ice
- ½ C frozen raspberries
- 1 C kale

Directions:

I. Add all of your ingredients to your blender or food processor and blend for about 30 seconds on high until smooth
II. Serve

Green Spice Smoothie

Ingredients:
- 1 C coconut water
- ¼ avocado
- 1 C baby spinach
- ½ C frozen blueberries
- 1 T chia seeds
- ½ T coconut oil
- ¼ tsp. chili powder
- ½ T honey
- 1 T shredded coconut flakes

Directions:

I. Add all of your ingredients to your blender or food processor and blend for about 30 seconds on high until smooth
II. Serve

Mint Chip Smoothie

Ingredients:
- 1 C coconut milk
- ½ avocado
- 1 T cacao nibs
- 1 serving protein powder (your preference of flavor)
- 1 tsp. honey

Directions:

I. Add all of your ingredients to your blender or food processor and blend for about 30 seconds on high until smooth
II. Serve

Psoriasis Treatment Smoothie

Ingredients:
- 1 C green tea
- 1/3 avocado
- 1 kiwi, skinned
- 1 C baby spinach
- 1/2 C blueberries
- 1 T chai seeds
- 1/2 tsp turmeric
- 1/2 tsp grated ginger
- 1/4 tsp cinnamon
- 1/2 T honey
- 1 C pitted cherries

Directions:

I. Add all of your ingredients to your blender or food processor and blend for about 30 seconds on high until smooth
II. Serve

Red Rose Smoothie

Ingredients:
- 1 C coconut water
- 1 C raspberries
- ½ C blueberries
- 1 prig rosemary, grated or chopped
- ½ T honey
- ice
- 1 C spinach
- 1 T cacao

Directions:

I. Add all of your ingredients to your blender or food processor and blend for about 30 seconds on high until smooth
II. Serve

Hot Fruit Smoothie

Ingredients:
- 1 C water
- ½ avocado
- ½ C strawberries
- 1 T flaxseed
- ¼ tsp. cayenne pepper
- ½ C raspberries
- 1 T cacao powder

Directions:

I. Add all of your ingredients to your blender or food processor and blend for about 30 seconds on high until smooth
II. Serve

Green Rose Smoothie

Ingredients:
- 1 C coconut water
- ½ C mango chunks
- 1 C spinach
- 1 tsp coconut oil
- honey
- rosemary sprigs
- ½ C mango chunks

Directions:
I. Add all of your ingredients to your blender or food processor and blend for about 30 seconds on high until smooth
II. Serve

Savory Banana Smoothie

Ingredients:
- 1 C almond milk
- 1 banana
- sage leaves
- honey
- ½ C blueberries
- ½ C mango chunks
- 1 C kale

Directions:

I. Add all of your ingredients to your blender or food processor and blend for about 30 seconds on high until smooth
II. Serve.

Anti-Bloat Smoothie

Ingredients:
- 1 C green
- 1/2 C blueberries
- 1/2 C papaya chunks
- 1/3 avocado
- 1 T chia seeds
- 1/2 tsp. turmeric
- 1/2 tsp ginger
- 1/4 tsp cayenne pepper
- 1 tsp honey
- 1 C baby spinach

Directions:

I. Add all of your ingredients to your blender or food processor and blend for about 30 seconds on high until smooth
II. Serve

Spicy Green Smoothie

Ingredients:
- 1 C coconut water
- 1 C baby spinach
- 1 banana
- ½ tsp coconut oil
- ¼ tsp cayenne pepper
- 1 T chia seeds

Directions:

I. Add all of your ingredients to your blender or food processor and blend for about 30 seconds on high until smooth
II. Serve

Strawberry Basil Smoothie

Ingredients:
- 1 C coconut water
- 1 banana
- ½ C strawberries
- ice
- mint leaves
- ¼ C greek yogurt

Directions:

I. Add all of your ingredients to your blender or food processor and blend for about 30 seconds on high until smooth
II. Serve

Red Mint Fruit Smoothie

Ingredients:
- 1 coconut water
- 1 banana
- 1 C fresh strawberries
- 1 C kale
- 1 T mint leaves
- 1 T flaxseed

Directions:

I. Add all of your ingredients to your blender or food processor and blend for about 30 seconds on high until smooth
II. Serve

Red Banana Smoothie

Ingredients:
- 1 C coconut water
- 1 banana
- ½ C strawberries
- mint leaves
- 1 T flaxseed

Directions:

I. Add all of your ingredients to your blender or food processor and blend for about 30 seconds on high until smooth
II. Serve

Turmeric Tot Smoothie

Ingredients:
- 1 C coconut water
- ½ avocado
- ½ C blueberries
- 1 spinach
- 1 T chia seeds

Directions:

I. Add all of your ingredients to your blender or food processor and blend for about 30 seconds on high until smooth
II. Serve

Turmeric Blast Smoothie

Ingredients:
- 1 C coconut water
- 1 apple, cored
- 1/3 banana
- 1/2 C blackberries
- 1/3 C bilberries
- 1 T oats
- 1 T macadamia nuts

Directions:

I. Add all of your ingredients to your blender or food processor and blend for about 30 seconds on high until smooth
II. Serve

Sunshine and Turmeric Smoothie

Ingredients;
- 1 C almond milk
- ½ C mango chinks
- 1 banana
- 1 T coconut oil
- ½ tsp turmeric
- ½ tsp cinnamon
- ½ tsp ginger
- salt
- ½ C pineapple chunks
- ½ T maca

Directions:

I. Add all of your ingredients to your blender or food processor and blend for about 30 seconds on high until smooth
II. Serve

Tropics Smoothie

Ingredients:
- ½ C water
- ½ C cilantro
- 1 C pineapple chunks
- ½ C mango chunks
- lime juice
- ¼ avocado

Directions:

I. Add all of your ingredients to your blender or food processor and blend for about 30 seconds on high until smooth
II. Serve

Turmeric and Chia Smoothie

Ingredients:
- 1 C coconut milk
- ½ avocado
- ½ C blueberries
- ½ tsp ginger
- ½ T honey
- 1 T chia seeds

Directions:

I. Add all of your ingredients to your blender or food processor and blend for about 30 seconds on high until smooth
II. Serve